OXFORD AMERICAN POCKET NOTES

Safe Opioid Prescribing for Nurse Practitioners

This material is not intended to be, and should not be considered, a substitute for medical or other professional advice. Treatment for the conditions described in this material is highly dependent on the individual circumstances. While this material is designed to offer accurate information with respect to the subject matter covered and to be current as of the time it was written, research and knowledge about medical and health issues is constantly evolving, and dose schedules for medications are being revised continually, with new side effects recognized and accounted for regularly. Readers must therefore always check the product information and clinical procedures with the most up-to-date published product information and data sheets provided by the manufacturers and the most recent codes of conduct and safety regulation. Oxford University Press and the authors make no representations or warranties to readers, express or implied, as to the accuracy or completeness of this material, including without limitation that they make no representations or warranties as to the accuracy or efficacy of the drug dosages mentioned in the material. The authors and the publishers do not accept, and expressly disclaim, any responsibility for any liability, loss, or risk that may be claimed or incurred as a consequence of the use and/or application of any of the contents of this material.

The Publisher is responsible for author selection and the Publisher and the Author(s) make all editorial decisions, including decisions regarding content. The Publisher and the Author(s) are not responsible for any product information added to this publication by companies purchasing copies of it for distribution to clinicians.

DISCLOSURES

Yvonne D'Arcy has received honoraria from Endo Pharmaceuticals, Pfizer, Ortho-McNeil, and Forrest Pharmaceuticals. She has also served on the Speakers Bureau for Pfizer and receives book royalties from HCPro.

Patricia Bruckenthal has provided consulting services for Ameritox Ltd, Cephalon, and Endo Pharmaceuticals.

O A P N
OXFORD AMERICAN POCKET NOTES

Safe Opioid Prescribing for Nurse Practitioners

Yvonne D'Arcy, MS, CRNP, CNS
Pain Medicine and Palliative Care Nurse Practitioner
Suburban Hospital
Johns Hopkins Medicine
Bethesda, Maryland

Patricia Bruckenthal, PhD, RN, ANP-C
Clinical Associate Professor
Stony Brook University School of Nursing
Stony Brook, New York

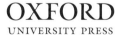

OXFORD
UNIVERSITY PRESS

Oxford University Press, Inc., publishes works that further
Oxford University's objective of excellence
in research, scholarship, and education.

Oxford New York

Auckland Cape Town Dar es Salaam Hong Kong Karachi
Kuala Lumpur Madrid Melbourne Mexico City Nairobi
New Delhi Shanghai Taipei Toronto

With offices in
Argentina Austria Brazil Chile Czech Republic France Greece
Guatemala Hungary Italy Japan Poland Portugal Singapore
South Korea Switzerland Thailand Turkey Ukraine Vietnam

Copyright © 2011 by Oxford University Press, Inc.

Published by Oxford University Press, Inc.
198 Madison Avenue, New York, New York 10016
www.oup.com

Oxford is a registered trademark of Oxford University Press

All rights reserved. No part of this publication may be reproduced,
stored in a retrieval system, or transmitted, in any form or by any
means, electronic, mechanical, photocopying, recording, or
otherwise, without the prior permission of Oxford Univers ity Press.

ISBN: 978-0-19-973770-3

9 8 7 6 5 4 3 2 1
Printed in China
on acid-free paper

**SAFE OPIOID PRESCRIBING
FOR NURSE PRACTITIONERS**

TABLE OF CONTENTS

I. Issues Surrounding Safe Prescribing 1

Treating Chronic Pain with Opioids 1

Legal Considerations 3

The Need for an Adequate Knowledge Base 7

II. Assessment: How to Determine if the Pain Complaint Needs Opioid Therapy 8

The Brief Pain Impact Questionnaire (BPIQ) 8

Criteria for Implementing Opioid Therapy 10

III. Screening for Opioid Risk 11

IV. Prescribing Opioids for Chronic Pain 13

Addiction, Dependency, Tolerance, and Pseudoaddiction 21

Opioid Prescriptions 24

Commonly Prescribed Opioids and Equivalent Doses 25

Medications for Mild Pain 26

Medications for Moderate Pain 26

Medications for Severe Pain 28

Extended-Release Medications 29

Opioid Rotation 34

Adjusting Opioids for the Older Patient 41

Using Opioids in Patients with a History of Substance Abuse 43

Treating Opioid-Related Side Effects 43

V. Developing a Comprehensive Treatment and Monitoring Plan 43

Appropriate Diagnosis 45

Psychological Assessment with Risk Assessment 45

Develop Treatment Plan 45

Informed Consent 46

Opioid Treatment Agreement 47

Consent for Chronic Opioid Therapy 48

Urine Drug Testing 51

Reassessment 61

Unmet Treatment Goals and Exit Strategy 66

Documentation 67

VI. Integrating Complementary Methods into the Treatment Plan 67

Questions to Consider for Complementary and Alternative Medicine Use 68

Notes 69

References 69

SAFE OPIOID PRESCRIBING FOR NURSE PRACTITIONERS

FOREWORD

Prescriptive authority is a major component of nurse practitioner practice. Most nurse practitioners are comfortable writing prescriptions for the medical management of chronic conditions such as hypertension or diabetes. However, when opioids are a part of the care plan, prescribing becomes more of a challenge and a concern.

In a survey of 400 nurse practitioners from primary care settings, hospitals, and specialty clinics, the respondents indicated that their basic nurse practitioner education did not prepare them to assess (62%), or treat (44%) long-term or persistant chronic pain. If the patient was using opioids short term, 73% of the respondents felt comfortable prescribing opioids to treat pain, but when the time frame was extended to 12 months or more, the comfort level with continuing to prescribe opioids fell to 32% (D'Arcy, 2009). This change in comfort level was in part caused by fear of regulatory oversight and the fear of causing addiction to opioid analgesics.

With a limited number of pain specialists available to help treat persistent chronic pain, it is important for nurse practitioners who are treating these patients to know how to prescribe opioid analgesic medications safely. The techniques and tools described in this book will help the nurse practitioner whose patients require opioid analgesics to feel safer and more confident as a prescriber.

Bill McCarberg, MD
Founder, Chronic Pain Management Program
Kaiser Permanente

and

Adjunct Assistant Clinical Professor
University of California, San Diego
San Diego, California

SAFE OPIOID PRESCRIBING FOR NURSE PRACTITIONERS

I. ISSUES SURROUNDING SAFE PRESCRIBING

There are a wide variety of issues surrounding the use and prescribing of opioid medications. Not only do prescribers need to know which opioid is most appropriate for a patient's pain complaint, but they also need to have a broad understanding of this class of medications and have confidence in their prescribing decisions. This component of prescribing is colored by issues, about legal and regulatory issues, especially when treating chronic pain. These pertinent concerns about safe prescribing will be addressed in the following sections of this clinical guide.

Treating Chronic Pain with Opioids

Patients with chronic, also called persistent, pain make up a large percentage of the patients seen in primary care settings. Many of these patients require opioid analgesics to achieve adequate control of their pain. There are also a significant number of opioid-dependent patients with chronic pain who are seen in acute care for surgery, trauma, or other injuries. Using opioid medications to control pain in these patients may challenge the comfort level of prescribing clinicians who are not familiar with using this class of drugs. The resultant undertreatment of pain can cause adverse outcomes to patients and negatively affect a patient's quality of life. Using safe prescribing practices can help to ensure the best outcomes for both patient and prescriber.

What constitutes safe prescribing? To prescribe controlled substances such as opioids in a safe manner, the healthcare provider should:

- Be aware of all the requirements for a legal prescription in their licensing state
- Use national guideline information and recommendations to guide practice

- Perform a complete and thorough history and physical examination to establish a diagnosis and treatment plan
- Screen patients for opioid risk and use treatment strategies that mitigate risk of misuse and assist in adherence.

Many national organizations recognize the use of opioids as a crucial component to providing adequate pain relief for patients. These are included in their guidelines and consensus statements:

- Veterans Health Administration/Department of Defense[1] recommends the use of appropriate opioid therapy to provide the best level of pain relief with the fewest side effects at the lowest effective dose. In addition, it recommends the development of a comprehensive treatment plan that includes monitoring for diversion when opioid analgesics are indicated for pain management.
- American Society of Anesthesiologists (ASA, 1997)[2] recommends the use of a multimodal treatment plan that includes medications of different types, including opioid analgesics.
- American Pain Society (APS, 2009)[3] Pat noted that the references are redundant here (both APA and AMA). However, I think in this case, they are helpful in indicating how current the guidelines are and can be kept as is provides practice recommendations when opioids are used for chronic non-cancer-related pain.
- American Society of Interventional Pain Physicians (ASIPP, 2008)[4] recommends the use of opioids for short-term pain relief but finds the evidence for long-term use is variable.
- A consensus statement by the American Academy of Pain Medicine (AAPM) and the APS (1997)[5] notes that accepted principles of practice when opioids are used should be considered a part of professional practice.

- A consensus statement by the AAPM, the APS, and the American Society of Addiction Medicine (ASAM, 2004)[6] finds that opioids should be considered as a component of an effective treatment plan for pain management after appropriate assessment.
- The American Geriatric Society (AGS, 2009)[7] has published a guideline with pharmacological recommendations for treating pain in older patients that includes opioid analgesics under certain circumstances.

Opioid prescribing is supported by national organizations and patient advocacy groups. It is incumbent on prescribers to understand how opioids should be prescribed and what the national recommendations are when long-term opioid treatment is being considered.

Legal Considerations

In many practices, opioid therapy will be a part of a daily prescribing regimen for select patients. Some practitioners are reluctant to prescribe opioids because they feel that when a patient needs chronic opioid therapy there is a high potential for creating addiction in that patient. In reality, there seems to be less of a risk than practitioners realize.

An analysis of studies on addiction in patients with chronic pain who were using opioids for a variety of pain conditions found that rates of addiction in these patients were similar to the general population.[8] In a study with 800 primary care patients who were using long-term opioid therapy, the rate of addiction was found to be between 4% and 6%.[9] In another study of patients on long-term opioid therapy the rate of addiction was 0.19% for patients who had never previously used opioids and 3.27% for patients who had used opioids in the past.[10] This indicates that roughly 95% of all patients who were taking opioids long term did not become addicted.

Nurse practitioners in the United States have had prescriptive authority for over 20 years. Each state has a different set of regulations related to the extent of this authority. Many states allow nurse practitioners to prescribe opioids in the Schedule II classification but other states limit prescriptive ability to Schedule III or lower. Nurse practitioners are bound by the tenets of the Controlled Substance Act (CSA), and prescribing is allowed only after the U.S. Drug Enforcement Administration (DEA) issues a license to prescribe controlled substances in the practitioners state of licensure. The rationale for including a drug in a particular Schedule Class was originally based on what was believed to be the medications, potential for abuse. This does not hold true today, as potential for abuse is dependent on many factors and may vary by geographic region, availability of supply, and cultural trends. Examples of Scheduled medications:

- Schedule I: drugs with high potential for abuse and no accepted medical use for treatment in the United States; lack of safety for use of the drug; ecstasy, heroin, LSD.
- Schedule II: drugs with high potential for abuse with a current medical use for treatment accepted in the United States; use may lead to severe physical or psychological dependence; cocaine, methadone, oxycodone and oxycodone combinations, morphine, fentanyl.
- Schedule III: drugs with less potential for abuse than those drugs in Schedules I and II; currently accepted medical use in the United States; moderate or low risk of physical or psychological dependence; anabolic steroids, buprenorphine, hydrocodone combinations, ketamine, nalorphine.
- Schedule IV: low potential for abuse compared to drugs in Schedule III; currently accepted medical use in the United States; the potential for physical dependence or psychological

dependence is limited compared to the drugs in Schedule III; alprazolam, diazepam, lorazepam, modafinil, pentazocine/nalaxone, sibutramine, eszopiclone.

- Schedule V: low potential for abuse compared to drugs listed in Schedule IV; currently accepted medical use in the United States; limited physical or psychological dependence relative to the substances listed in Schedule IV; guaifenesin/codeine, atropine/difenoxin.

The primary federal control for opioid prescribing is regulated by the U.S. Food and Drug Administration (FDA) and the DEA. The CSA of 1970 gives the DEA primary control over prescribing policies for controlled substances; setting production quotas; and regulating prescribers, dispensing pharmacies, manufacturers, distributors, importers, and researchers in activities involving opioid analgesics. As an arm of the federal government, the DEA plays an important role in enforcing compliance with these laws.

Since each states governs what drugs a nurse practitioner can prescribe, the state-level regulations reflect the CSA and individualize the practice for the state. In addition, some states, such as California, have enacted Intractable Pain Treatment Acts that help to identify patients who are potential candidates for opioid analgesics thus making clinicians more comfortable with opioid prescribing. They define intractable pain and the conditions that apply when opioids are being prescribed. These Acts also define the use and limits of disciplinary action related to opioid prescribing.

Despite practitioners' fears, regulatory sanction and oversight is rare. A recent survey of 963,385 MDs indicated that adequate documentation in medical records reduces the risk of legal action against prescribers to very small.[8] In the same group, when records from 2003 and 2004 were reviewed, they indicated 47 arrests and 53 DEA revocations.[8] A lack of primary patient-physician relationship was cited as a common cause of prescribing violations. Without a patient-physician relationship, continued opioid prescribing cannot be supported. Other reasons for legal actions included:

- Prescriber substance abuse
- Fraud
- Prescribing despite loss of medical license
- Sex in exchange for prescriptions
- Prescribing without seeing the patient[8]

Most states in conjunction with the federal government govern the regulations for the prescribing of opioids. Many states also track prescriptions for opioids and opioid prescribers via state prescription monitoring programs. In the larger picture, in the United States in 2002, only 120 prescribers were sanctioned by State Medical Boards, and many of these practitioners had multiple violations.[8]

From the patient's perspective, the lack of adequate pain management is providing a means of raising awareness of the effects of inadequate pain relief. For example, in the *Estate of Henry James v. Hillhaven*, after the death of the patient, the estate was awarded $1.5 million in compensatory damages for inadequate pain control. The patient's pain was well controlled using opioid analgesics while he was hospitalized. Upon transfer, the admitting nurse in a skilled nursing facility was held liable for citing the patient as addicted to opioid medication and subsequently substituting an alternate medication for some of the morphine doses. The patient's family sued for damages as a result of pain and suffering from inadequate pain management.

In other cases, California elder abuse laws were used to hold prescribers liable for discharging patients with high pain scores from their service and not adequately providing pain control.[11,12] In one case, a medical practitioner was required to attend pain management education courses and was cited by the state medical board for inadequate pain relief.[11,12]

Taken together, both fear of regulatory oversight and lack of understanding of the characteristics of opioids can lead to inadequate pain management.

The Need for an Adequate Knowledge Base

Treating patients with opioid analgesics requires a specific knowledge of how these medications act pharmacologically. In a survey of 400 nurse practitioners, the respondents indicated that their comfort level with opioid prescribing was good for short-term use (73%), but once pain became a chronic problem (longer than 12 months), the comfort level for prescribing opioids fell to 32%.[13] When asked to rank barriers to opioid prescribing, fear of addiction and concern about increased regulatory oversight were ranked second and third out of 5 possible responses.[13] Some of these concerns may be based on the fact that approximately 50% of the respondents indicated that their basic nurse practitioner education did not prepare them to assess and treat chronic pain or select the correct medications for chronic pain.[13]

Healthcare providers who prescribe opioids should be knowledgeable about the medications, correct doses, and adverse effects. Perscriptions for opioids should be specifically written to avoid opportunities for diversion. A safely written prescription includes:

- Medical record documentation of a risk/benefit ratio analysis before a medication is prescribed for a patient to

determine if the suggested treatment is the best option for the condition
- A prior patient assessment using screening tools and diagnostic evaluation to help determine if the medication is a safe choice for the patient
- A clear, readable prescription with clear directions for use
- The dosage and directions in long hand when feasible (ten mg versus 10 mg)
- The right drug in the right dose for the right patient[16]

Using national guidelines recommendations, expert pain specialist referrals, and becoming knowledgeable about opioids will help practitioners make the correct decisions when opioids are being prescribed.

II. ASSESSMENT: HOW TO DETERMINE IF THE PAIN COMPLAINT WARRENTS OPIOID THERAPY

Assessment is the key to correct medication selection. The most commonly used pain assessment scale is the Numeric Rating Scale (NRS), which rates pain intensity on a 0-to-10 scale, where 0 equals no pain and 10 equals the worst pain imaginable. This scale is useful in measuring medication efficacy, but for chronic pain more comprehensive assessment is needed.

The Brief Pain Impact Questionnaire (BPIQ)

A pain intensity rating such as the 0-to-10 numeric pain scale may not provide enough information to determine if opioid analgesics are an appropriate treatment choice. Using a structured questionnaire format such as the Brief Pain Impact Questionnaire (BPIQ) can help nurse practitioners and other clinicians ensure that a more comprehensive assessment, including salient information about the pain complaint and co-existing health concerns, is addressed in the care plan (See Table 1). Not only does this questionnaire pinpoint the effect of the pain on the patient's lifestyle, but it also provides a means of assessing overall daily function, which may be a better measure of pain management than a numeric pain rating.

Table 1 Brief Pain Impact Questionnaire (BPIQ)
- How strong is your pain, right now, worst/average over the past week?
- How many days over the past week have you been unable to do what you would like to do because of your pain?
- Over the past week, how often has pain interfered with your ability to take care of yourself, for example with bathing, eating, dressing and going to the toilet?
- Over the past week, how often has pain interfered with your ability to take care of your home-related chores such as grocery shopping, preparing meals, paying bills, and driving?
- How often do you participate in pleasurable activities such as hobbies, socializing with friends, and travel? Over the past week how often has pain interfered with these activities?
- How often do you do some type of exercise? Over the past week, how often has pain interfered with your ability to exercise?
- Does pain interfere with your ability to think clearly?
- Does pain interfere with your appetite? Have you lost weight?
- Does pain interfere with your sleep? How often over the last week?
- Has pain interfered with your energy, mood, personality, or relationships with other people?
- Over the past week have you taken pain medications?
- Has your use of alcohol or other drugs ever caused a problem for you or those close to you?
- How would you rate your health at the present time?
From Weiner DK, Herr K, Rudy TE (Eds), *Persistent Pain in Older Adults: An Interdisciplinary Guide for Treatment.* Reproduced with the permission of Springer Publishing Company, LLC, New York, NY 10036.

Criteria for Implementing Opioid Therapy

A healthcare provider who is considering using opioids as part of a pain management plan should use certain criteria to determine the suitability of this option for the individual patient. Adhering to recommended criteria will also ensure that using opioids for a particular patient provides more benefit than risk. The APS and AAPM opioid treatment guidelines for selecting a patient for opioid therapy include:

- Before starting chronic opioid therapy, the healthcare provider should conduct a complete history and physical examination and an assessment of risk of substance abuse, misuse, or addiction.
- Identify if there are co-morbid conditions that would preclude using non-opioid analgesics such as peptic ulcer disease or liver disease.
- Healthcare providers should consider using a trial of chronic opioid therapy if the pain is moderate to severe, if non-opioid choices are contraindicated, if the pain is adversely affecting the patient's quality of life or ability to function, or if the benefit/risk analysis indicates more benefit than risk for the patient.
- Documentation should include baseline information on the risk/benefit assessment, history and physical, and diagnostic testing, and the documentation should be done on an ongoing basis.[3]

Risk assessment and risk stratification can be done using screening tools listed in the next section. There are some important elements of selecting opioid therapy for an individual patient with a specific pain condition:

- For some conditions such as trigeminal neuralgia and other neuropathic conditions, a trial of chronic opioid therapy is indicated only if neuropathic medications such

as anticonvulsants have been tried and were not successful in bringing pain to an acceptable level.
- In patients with poorly defined pain conditions, patients with somatoform pain, or patients with legal issues related to the pain condition still pending, chronic opioid therapy is considered to be less successful.
- Efficacy for chronic opioid therapy is not well demonstrated in pain syndromes such as some types of low back pain, fibromyalgia, or daily headache.
- A personal or family history of alcohol or drug abuse is most predictive for drug abuse, misuse, or other aberrant drug-taking behaviors when chronic opioid therapy is used. Chronic opioid therapy, if used, would warrant stricter monitoring practices.
- Some research finds that younger patients and those with psychiatric conditions are more likely to demonstrate aberrant drug-taking behaviors.[3]

As always, the individual patient's needs should be considered when opioids are being initiated as a part of the comprehensive plan of care.

III. SCREENING FOR OPIOID RISK

Each patient seen by the nurse practitioner should have a comprehensive admission evaluation. For patients with pain, this includes an assessment of pain intensity, location, and duration; pain descriptors; and what makes the pain improve or worsen. It is not possible to tell from the patient's clinical presentation alone whether he or she will who may have difficulty managing chronic opioid therapy. Opioid risk screening tools can help determine who may have difficulty with opioids or who may develop aberrant drug-taking behaviors.

Relevant information about potential difficulties with opioid use requires assessment prior to initiating opioid therapy. Pertinent questions include history of any illicit substance use or any past history of difficulty using pain medications. If the patient has a positive answer to these questions, then the prescriber needs to gather specific information about drug type, dose, and length of illicit drug use. For those patients falling into the high-risk category, more frequent monitoring is required, as well as the use of non-opioid treatment options such as anesthesia-related blockade or injection, physical therapy, or psychological support. A team approach is needed for patients who are at high risk, and the team may consist of many types of practitioners. It is helpful to include a member who has expertise in treating patients with addictive disease.

Screening patients for risks of addiction, abuse, and misuse can help stratify patient risk and facilitate discussions about chronic opioid therapy between healthcare providers and patients.

Some of the simplest screening instruments are the CAGE and the TRAUMA screen. The CAGE questions are:

- Have you ever tried to **Cut** down on your alcohol or drug use?
- Have people **Annoyed** you by commenting on or critiquing your drinking or drug use?
- Have you ever felt bad or **Guilty** about your drinking or drug use?
- Have you ever needed an **"Eye opener"** first thing in the morning to steady your nerves or get rid of a hangover?

The higher the number of responses, the greater the likelihood that the patient has a drug or alcohol abuse problem.[3,18]

In the TRAUMA screen the person's injury profile is assessed. To perform this screen the patient is asked: Since your 18th birthday have you:

- Had any fractures or dislocations to your bones or joints (excluding sports injuries)?
- Been injured in a traffic accident?
- Injured your head (excluding sports injuries)?
- Been in a fight or assaulted while intoxicated?
- Been injured while intoxicated?

If the patient has a positive response to two of the questions in the TRAUMA screen, there is a high potential for abuse.[3] More formal screening tools include the SOAPP-R, ORT, DIRE, and COMM.

Using these screening tools as part of a comprehensive plan of care can help determine which patients may have more difficulty adhering to chronic opioid therapy and require closer monitoring. In turn, the healthcare provider can be more confident in prescribing opioids for most patients who have negative screens and be alert for those patients who may require more frequent screens. The level of risk can help guide decisions as to how closely and frequently opioid monitoring practices, such as pill counts and urine drug tests, should be employed.

IV. PRESCRIBING OPIOIDS FOR CHRONIC PAIN

For some patients with chronic pain, opioids will be a part of the plan of care. Learning to identify high-risk and low-risk patients with a tool such as the ORT will help prescribers feel more comfortable with the process. Learning the differences between addiction and dependency will also help

Screener and Opioid Assessment for Patients with Pain (SOAPP-R)

Assesses for abuse potential using a 24-item self-report measure. A reliable and valid measure, where a score equal to or greater than 18 indicates a high risk of misuse or abuse. Used as an initial screen.

	Never 0	Seldom 1	Sometimes 2	Often 3	Very Often 4
1. How often do you have mood swings?	☐	☐	☐	☐	☐
2. How often have you felt a need for higher doses of medication to treat your pain?	☐	☐	☐	☐	☐
3. How often have you felt impatient with your doctors?	☐	☐	☐	☐	☐
4. How often have you felt that things are just too overwhelming that you can't handle them?	☐	☐	☐	☐	☐
5. How often is there tension in the home?	☐	☐	☐	☐	☐
6. How often have you counted pain pills to see how many are remaining?	☐	☐	☐	☐	☐
7. How often have you been concerned that people will judge you for taking pain medication?	☐	☐	☐	☐	☐
8. How often do you feel bored?	☐	☐	☐	☐	☐

9. How often have you taken more pain medication than you were supposed to?	☐	☐	☐
10. How often have you worried about being left alone?	☐	☐	☐
11. How often have you felt a craving for medication?	☐	☐	☐
12. How often have others expressed concern over your use of medication?	☐	☐	☐
13. How often have any of your close friends had a problem with alcohol or drugs?	☐	☐	☐
14. How often have others told you that you had a bad temper?	☐	☐	☐
15. How often have you felt consumed by the need to get pain medication?	☐	☐	☐
16. How often have you run out of pain medication early?	☐	☐	☐
17. How often have others kept you from getting what you deserve?	☐	☐	☐
18. How often, in your lifetime, have you had legal problems or been arrested?	☐	☐	☐
19. How often have you attended an AA or NA meeting?	☐	☐	☐

(continued)

Screener and Opioid Assessment for Patients with Pain (SOAPP-R) (Continued)

	Never 0	Seldom 1	Sometimes 2	Often 3	Very Often 4
20. How often have you been in an argument that was so out of control that someone got hurt?	☐	☐	☐	☐	☐
21. How often have you been sexually abused?	☐	☐	☐	☐	☐
22. How often have others suggested that you have a drug or alcohol problem?	☐	☐	☐	☐	☐
23. How often have you had to borrow pain medications from your family or friends?	☐	☐	☐	☐	☐
24. How often have you been treated for an alcohol or drug problem?	☐	☐	☐	☐	☐

This table was published in Butler SF, Fernandez K, Benoit C, Budman SH, Jamison RN. Validation of the revised Screener and Opioid Assessment for Patients with Pain (SOAPP-R). *J Pain* 2008;9(4):360–372. Copyright Elsevier 2008.

SAFE OPIOID PRESCRIBING FOR NURSE PRACTITIONERS

Opioid Risk Tool (ORT)
Screens for aberrant behaviors in patients taking long-term opioids using a 5-item yes/no format self-report measure. Scores of 0 to 3 are considered low risk, 4 to 7 are considered moderate risk, and 8 and over are considered high risk. Has excellent ability to discriminate low-risk vs. high-risk patients, both male and female. Used when aberrant behaviors are suspected.

Item		Mark each box that applies	Item score if female	Item score if male
1.	Family history of substance abuse			
	Alcohol	[ ]	1	3
	Illegal drugs	[ ]	2	3
	Prescription drugs	[ ]	4	4
2.	Personal history of substance abuse			
	Alcohol	[ ]	3	3
	Illegal drugs	[ ]	4	4
	Prescription drugs	[ ]	5	5
3.	Age (mark box if 16–45)	[ ]	1	1
4.	History of preadolescent sexual abuse	[ ]	3	0
5.	Psychological disease Attention deficit disorder, obsessive-compulsive disorder, bipolar, schizophrenia, depression	[ ] [ ]	2 1	2 1

Total ORT Score (sum of 1–5)
Interpretation of ORT Score
Low risk (score of 0–3)
Moderate risk (score of 4–7)
High risk (score of 8 and above)

Reprinted with permission from Webster LR, Webster RM. Predicting aberrant behaviors in opioid-treated patients: preliminary validation of the Opioid Risk Tool. *Pain Med* 2005;6(6):432–442.

Diagnosis, Intractability, Risk and Efficacy Score (D.I.R.E.)

A clinician-rated scale with questions in four categories: diagnosis, intractability, risk, and efficacy. The categories are further divided into psychological, chemical health, reliability, and social support. A score of 14 and above indicates a patient is a good risk for opioid therapy. Patients with lower scores are not considered good risks for opioid therapy. Used for screening at the initiation of opioid therapy.

D.I.R.E. Score: Patient selection for chronic opioid analgesic
SCORE FACTOR

Diagnosis	1 = Benign chronic condition with minimal objective findings or not definite medical diagnosis (e.g., non-specific back pain).
	2 = Slowly progressive condition concordant with moderate pain or fixed condition with moderate objective findings (e.g., back pain with moderate degenerative changes).
	3 = Advanced condition concordant with severe pain with objective findings (e.g., severe ischemic vascular disease).
Intractability	1 = Few therapies have been tried and the patient takes a passive role in his/her pain management process.
	2 = Most customary treatments have been tried but the patient is not fully engaged in the pain management process.
	3 = Patient fully engaged in a spectrum of appropriate treatments but with inadequate response.
Risk **P**sychological	(**R** = Total of **P** + **C** + **R** + **S** below)
	1 = Serious personality dysfunction or mental illness interfering with care (e.g., severe personality disorder).
	2 = Personality or mental health interferes moderately (e.g., mild-moerate depression).
	3 = Good communication with clinic. No significant personality dysfunction.

Chemical health	1 = Active or very recent use of illicit drugs, excessive alcohol, or prescription drug abuse. 2 = Chemical coper (uses medications to cope with stress) or history of CD in remission. 3 = No CD history. Not drug-focused or chemically reliant.
Reliability	1 = History of numerous problems: medication misuse, missed appointments, rarely follows through. 2 = Occasional difficulties with compliance, but generally reliable. 3 = Highly reliable patient with meds, appointments, and treatment.
Social support	1 = Life in chaos. Little family support and few close relationships. Loss of most normal life roles. 2 = Reduction in some relationships and life roles. 3 = Supportive family/close relationships. Involved in work or school.
Efficacy score	1 = Poor function or minimal pain relief despite moderate to high doses. 2 = Moderate benefit with function improved in a number of ways (or insufficient information, for those who haven't yet tried opioid therapy or tried at a duration too short for legitimate trial). 3 = Good improvement in pain and function and quality of life with stable doses over time.

For each factor, rate the patient's score from 1–3 based on the explanations in the right-hand column.
Total score = D + I + R + E
Score 7–13: Not a suitable candidate for long-term opioid analgesia
Score 14–21: Good candidate for long-term opioid analgesia

This table was published in Belgrade MJ, Schamber CD, Lindgren BR. The DIRE Score: predicting outcomes of opioid prescribing for chronic pain. *J Pain* 2006;7(9):671–681. Copyright Elsevier 2006.

Current Opioid Misuse Measure (COMM)

A 17-item self-report measure to identify aberrant-drug related behaviors for patients on chronic opioid therapy. The COMM is a newer tool that can identify emotional/psychiatric issues, evidence of lying, appointment patterns, and medication misuse/noncompliance.[19,20] Used as an ongoing screen.

1. How often have you had trouble with thinking clearly or had memory problems?
2. How often do people complain that you are not completing necessary tasks (i.e., doing things that need to be done, such as going to class, work, or appointments)?
3. How often have you had to go to someone other than your prescribing physician to get sufficient pain relief from your medications (i.e., another doctor, the emergency room)?
4. How often have you taken your medications differently from how they are prescribed?
5. How often have you seriously thought about hurting yourself?
6. How much of your time was spent thinking about opioid medications (having enough, taking them, dosing schedule, etc.)?
7. How often have you been in an argument?
8. How often have you had trouble controlling your anger (e.g., road rage, screaming)?
9. How often have you needed to take pain medications belonging to someone else?
10. How often have you been worried about how you're handling your medications?
11. How often have others been worried about how you're handling your medications?
12. How often have you had to make an emergency phone call or show up at the clinic without an appointment?
13. How often have you gotten angry with people?
14. How often have you had to take more of your medication than prescribed?
15. How often have you borrowed pain medication from someone else?
16. How often have you used your pain medicine for symptoms other than for pain (e.g., to help you sleep, improve your mood, or relieve stress)?
17. How often have you had to visit the emergency room?

This table has been reproduced with permission of the International Association of the Study of Pain (IASP). The table may not be reproduced for any other purpose without permission. Butler SF, Budman SH, et al. Development and Validation of the Current Opioid Misuse Measure. *Pain* 2007; 130(1–2): 144–156.

prescribers understand just what conditions they're dealing with when they prescribe opioid medications.

In some instances the health care provider may be unaware of a history of addiction; in other cases, the information may be mentioned in the initial intake documentation by the prescriber. In the acute care setting, the health care provider may be called to see a patient with uncontrolled pain where addiction is playing a role in the level of pain medication requirements. For long-term therapy, the health care provider should always follow the recommendation for setting up a formal treatment agreement that includes information on addiction and dependency, and sets the requirements for compliance. Goal setting should include acceptable levels of pain intensity and level of function, among other mutually agreed upon goals. If the patient fails to progress toward the goals of care, the prescriber may eliminate the opioid prescribing portion of care and continue with options that do not include opioid analgesics. Risk assessment tools can help determine which patients may require more frequent monitoring and urine screens. The following sections will give additional information on how to assess and stratify patients for monitoring strategies.

Addiction, Dependency, Tolerance, and Pseudoaddiction
Before prescribing opioids, it is important to understand the meaning of *addiction*, *tolerance, dependency*, and *pseudoaddiction*. Some prescribers observe behaviors that they believe indicate addiction when in fact they may be a demonstration of undertreated pain or tolerance. The following definitions will help to clarify the difference between addiction and dependence and what types of behaviors are more predictive of addiction.

Addiction is based on the "4 C's":

- Craving for the favored substance
- Compulsive use
- Lack of control over the drug
- Continued use despite harm

By definition, addiction is a chronic neurobiological disease with genetic, psychosocial, and environmental factors influencing its development and manifestations.[21,22] In general, addiction is uncommon in most practices, but some patients who exhibit aberrant behaviors are seen as addicted and many of these patients are overlabeled and undertreated. Aberrant behaviors will be discussed in a later section of this book. Addicts tend to misuse all types of substances and, in addition to oral misuse, can inject, snort, or smoke oral or other opioids to get the euphoric effect they are seeking.

Dependency is an entirely different category than addiction. It is defined as a state of adaptation that is manifested by a drug class-specific withdrawal syndrome that can be produced by:

- Abrupt cessation
- Rapid dose reduction
- Decreasing blood levels of the drug and/or administration of an antagonist[22]

Patients who are dependent on opioids to relieve their pain should not be labeled as addicts. The pain relief afforded from the use of opioids allows these patients to maintain relationships and increase their level of function. It is, however, a fact, based on physiological adaptation to the medication, that all addicts are dependent on their opioid substances. Conversely, few patients who take opioids regularly develop the disease of addiction from these medications.

Tolerance is not a sign of addiction; it is merely a lessening of the medication effect that takes place over time.[22] This effect can be related to pain relief, but it can also refer to side effects such as sedation or nausea. The only opioid side effect that a patient will not become tolerant to is constipation, so a bowel regime should be part of the treatment plan for all patients on chronic opioid therapy. True tolerance to opioid medication is not a common occurrence. If a patient describes a lessening of analgesic effect to a previously effective opioid regime, worsening of pain condition, a new pain problem, or a psychosocial problem, the cause should be explored.

Pseudoaddiction is really a sign of undertreated pain. Perceived drug-seeking behaviors such as clock watching will disappear if the patient is provided with adequate analgesia.

Understanding Aberrant Behaviors

Some patients who are taking opioids regularly to manage chronic pain can develop aberrant behaviors that may or may not indicate addiction. Some behaviors that are less predictive of addiction include hoarding medications, taking someone else's medication, requesting a specific drug or dose, raising drug doses without a prescription several times, drinking more alcohol when in pain, smoking cigarettes to relieve pain, and using opioids to treat other symptoms. These behaviors may be exhibited for reasons not related to addiction. They may stem from unrelieved pain related to undertreatment, or financial concerns. Some behaviors seem to be more serious and have more severe consequences. Behaviors that are more predictive of addiction include concurrent use of illicit drugs, stealing or selling prescription drugs, injecting oral medications, repeated resistance to changes in therapy although there are clear negative effects, and deterioration in family and work relationships related to drug use.[23]

Opioid Prescriptions

Prescribing opioids for chronic pain begins with an understanding of the elements of a prescription and the criteria for a safe prescription. There are certain elements that all prescriptions need to have to be legal documents. A safe prescription for opioids must contain:

- Date of issue
- Patient's name and address
- Practitioner's name, address, and DEA registration number
- Drug name, strength, dosage form
- Quantity prescribed
- Directions for use
- Number of refills authorized
- Manual signature of prescriber[24]

Prescribers should never pre-sign or post-date prescriptions for other staff to fill in, predate prescriptions, or prescribe for patients with whom they do not have a prescriber-patient relationship. When prescribing opioids, healthcare providers should consider the following criteria to ensure that the prescription they are providing will be the best option for the patient and to provide adequate information for documentation:

- The practitioner performs and documents a risk/benefit ratio analysis before a medication is prescribed for a patient.

- Opioid risk screening tools are used to help determine if the medication is a safe choice for the patient.
- The prescription is clear and readable, with clear directions for use.
- The right drug is prescribed in the right dose for the right patient.[25]

Commonly Prescribed Opioids and Equivalent Doses

There are variety of short-acting, combination, and extended-release opioids. Choice of opioid may be related to type, duration, and intensity of pain among other reasons. One method to classify medications is the World Health Organization Ladder.

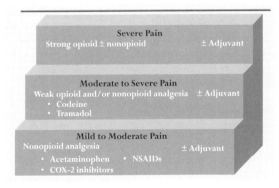

Figure 1 WHO Step Approach to Cancer Pain.
COX = cyclooxygenase; NSAID = nonsteroidal anti-inflammatory drugs
Source: World Health Organization (WHO).

Medications for Mild Pain
Acetaminophen
- Maximum daily dose 4,000 mg, to include amounts found in combination medications such as hydrocodone with acetaminophen, or oxycodone with acetaminophen
- Use caution with patients who have liver dysfunction or who consume alcohol regularly.

Nonsteroidal Anti-inflammatory Drugs (NSAIDs)
NONSELECTIVE MEDICATIONS

Ibuprofen, naproxen, and ketoprofen are used for mild pain alone or can be used with opioids for added analgesic effect.

SELECTIVE COX-2 INHIBITORS

Celecoxib (Celebrex) spares the prostaglandin lining of the stomach. It can be used alone or in combination with opioids for added analgesic effect.

NEW ADDITIONS TO THE DRUG CLASS

Targeted peripheral formulation of NSAIDs decrease pain in specific areas such as joints and have a very low potential for systemic uptake. Examples: ketoprofen gel 1%, diclofenac sodium (Pennsaid) liquid, ketoprofen patch (Flector).

Medications for Moderate Pain
Short-Acting Combination Medications for Intermittent Pain, Breakthrough Pain

CODEINE-CONTAINING MEDICATIONS
- Codeine, Tylenol #3 (codeine 30 mg combined with acetaminophen 325 mg)
- Codeine has a high profile for side effects such as constipation and gastrointestinal disturbances (nausea and vomiting).[26,27]

- Often used as a component in cough syrups as a cough suppressant[28]
- Has an elixir form, which is convenient for patients who have difficulty swallowing pills or for use with enteral feeding tubes
- Use caution in breastfeeding women: they may inadvertently give their infants a morphine overdose if they are ultra-rapid codeine metabolizers.[28]

Hydrocodone-Containing Medications

- Examples: Vicodin, Lortab, Norco, Lortab elixir
- Designed to be used for moderate pain
- Many patients tolerate these medications very well for intermittent pain or for breakthrough pain.
- Elixir form is very effective and can be used with patients who have difficulty swallowing pills or with enteral feeding tubes

Oxycodone-Containing Medications

- Examples: Oxycodone, Percocet, Roxicet, Percodan, Oxyfast
- Designed for treating moderate pain
- To help alleviate nausea, giving the medication with milk or after meals is recommended.[28]

Oxymorphone-Containing Medications

- Opana is a medication designed to treat moderate to severe pain.
- Has a more extended half-life than other medications of the same class, resulting in a decreased need for breakthrough medications.[29,30]
- Should be taken 1 hour before or 2 hours after a meal.[28]
- Also available in an injectable form for use during labor (Numorphan).[27,28]

Tramadol (Ultram, Ultracet)
- Combination of a mu agonist, opioid-like medication, and SSRI (selective serotonin reuptake inhibitor) type of medication[27]
- Designed for use with moderate pain
- Doses should be reduced for patients with increased creatinine levels, patients with cirrhosis, and older patients.
- May increase the risk for seizures and serotonin syndrome[28]
- Patients should be instructed to taper off the medication gradually when discontinuing the medication.
- It should not be stopped suddenly.[28]

Tapentadol (Nucynta)
- A new combination medication with a formulation similar to tramadol
- It is a centrally acting medication designed for use in moderate to severe pain.
- It is a medication combining mu agonist action and a norepinephrine reuptake inhibitor.
- This combined action gives the medication added analgesic effect.

Medications for Severe Pain
Hydromorphone (Dilaudid)
- An extremely potent analgesic designed for use with severe pain
- Commonly used after the usual medications for pain (e.g., Vicodin and Percocet) are unsuccessful
- Because of the strength of this medication, it is possible to give small amounts and get good pain relief with fewer side effects.
- A new extended-release formulation Exalgo was recently released.

Morphine
- Examples: Immediate-release morphine (MSIR), Roxanol elixir
- The gold standard for pain relief
- The standard for equianalgesic conversions and has a long history of use in many different forms for pain control
- Indicated for severe pain
- The biggest drawback to morphine is the side effect profile: constipation, nausea/vomiting, delirium, and hallucinations are some of the most commonly reported adverse effects.

Fentanyl Transmucosal
- Sublimaze, Actiq, Fentora, Onsolis
- There is no oral pill formulation possible for fentanyl. The route of administration is either transdermal or buccal.
- For breakthrough pain in opioid-tolerant patients, the transmucosal medications can be rubbed across the buccal membrane and absorbed directly into the cardiac circulation.
- The fast absorption makes this medication a risk for oversedation. Thus, it should be used only for breakthrough pain in opioid-tolerant cancer patients or patients with chronic pain who take opioid medications on a daily basis.
- These medications are not meant to be used for acute or postoperative pain[28] and should not be used in opioid-naïve patients since serious oversedation can occur.[23]

Extended-Release Medications
For patients with persistent pain, extended-release medications can provide a consistent blood level of medication that can provide a steady comfort level. This may increase functionality and improve quality of life, enhance sleep, and allow the patient to participate in meaningful daily activities.

Extended-release medications usually have a slower onset of action (30 to 90 minutes) with a relatively long duration of action (up to 72 hours).[31]

When a patient has pain that lasts throughout the day, is taking short-acting medications, and has reached the maximum dose limitations of the non-opioid medication, the prescriber should consider switching the patient to an extended-release or long-acting medication. Some of the short-acting medications have an extended-release (ER) formulation (e.g., Vicodin ER, Opana ER, Ultram ER, OxyContin, Kadian, Avinza, Embeda, MS Contin, and Exalgo). Most are pure mu agonist medications, such as morphine, with an ER action that allows the medication to dissolve slowly in the gastrointestinal tract. Some ER medications are encapsulated into beads that allow gastric secretions to enter the bead and force the medication out. Other ER formulations have a coating around an ER plasticized compound that keeps the medication from dissolving too quickly.

When an ER medication is being started, the patient should be instructed as follows:

- ER medications of all types should never be broken, chewed, or degraded in any way to enhance the absorption of the medications. Doing so runs the risk of all the medication being given at one time, and there is a high risk for potentially fatal oversedation.
- The exception to this is Kadian and Avinza which are capsules that can be opened and the encapsulated beads sprinkled onto food such as applesauce to facilitate swallowing.
- Most ER medications should not be taken with alcohol. Doing so degrades the ER mechanism and allows for faster absorption of the medication, which can cause potentially fatal oversedation.

- ER medications should not be injected.
- ER medications should not be crushed and inserted into enteral feeding tubes.
- ER medications should not be used on an as-needed basis; rather, they should be taken as scheduled daily doses.[26]
- If the patient experiences end-of-dose failure several hours before the next dose of medication is due, the interval should be shortened or the dose should be increased.[26]

When converting a patient from short-acting medications, the health care provider should follow these rules of thumb:

- If the medication is the same compound (Percocet to OxyContin, for example), equivalent 24 hour total doses of the medication can be prescribed but the dosing interval adjusted for the ER.
- If the medication is a different drug (Percocet to MS Contin, for example), the daily dose should be calculated using the equianalgesic conversion table and reduced, usually by 30%. To ensure that adequate pain relief is maintained, additional doses of breakthrough medication should be prescribed: about 5% to 15% of the total daily dose to be taken every 2 hours as needed.[26]

Methadone
- Examples: Dolophine, Methadose
- Methadone is considered to be a long-acting medication because it has an extended half-life of 15 to 60 hours.[26]
- However, pain relief from the oral form may only last at 4 to 6 hours.[28]
- Dosing must be done very carefully to avoid oversedating the patient, which may become apparent only a day or two after the doses are given due to the long half-life of this medication.

- Dose escalation should be done no more often than every 3 to 7 days.[26]
- Methadone can be prescribed legally by general practitioners in primary care for pain relief. This indication for pain control must be written on the prescription.
- The current recommendation of the APS is that only pain management practitioners or those skilled and knowledgeable about methadone should prescribe the drug.[26,32]

An additional risk factor for this medication is the potential for QTc interval prolongation and, with higher doses, torsades de pointes. Primary care providers are advised to obtain a baseline ECG for patients who are taking daily methadone and should obtain regular ECGs as the doses escalate to above 100 mg/day.[26,A]

Fentanyl Patches
- Example: Duragesic
- This is the only transdermal opioid application that is available for use in a delivery system that contains a specified dose of fentanyl in a gel formulation.
- Designed for use with opioid-tolerant patients and should never be used for acute pain or with opioid-naïve patients
- The medication effect begins as the medication depot develops in the subcutaneous fat; it can take 12 to 18 hours for pain relief to begin.[27,32]
- It can also take up to 48 hours for steady-state blood levels to develop, so when the patch is being started, the patient will need additional breakthrough pain medication to control pain.[32]

- The patch should never be cut and heat should not be applied over the patch, since this can cause increased medication delivery.
- The patch should be disposed of in a closed container to avoid the possibility of someone who is not opioid-tolerant using the patch, with resultant overdose.[32]
- To convert to a 25-microgram fentanyl patch, the patient should be taking one of the following: 30 mg oxycodone per day for 2 weeks, 8 mg hydromorphone per day for 2 weeks, or 60 mg oral morphine per day for 2 weeks.[B]

New Tamper Resistant Extended-Release Medications

Morphine Sulfate Combined with Naltrexone Hydrochloride (Embeda)

- Used for moderate to severe pain
- Should be used for opioid-tolerant patients only
- Morphine is part of the outer pellet with a naltrexone center, so pellets should never be crushed or chewed since the result could be a naltrexone-induced withdrawal syndrome.

Hydromorphone HCL (Exalgo)

- Used for around-the-clock pain relief for opioid-tolerant patients
- For moderate to severe pain that is expected to last an extended period
- Recently approved for use

Opioid Prescribing Summary

Opioid medications are easily metabolized by the body. They provide excellent pain relief and can be used in combination with other medications, such as antidepressants or NSAIDs. Opioids bind to mu receptors in the central nervous system to produce analgesia. Recently there has been evidence to suggest genetic differences in opioid binding sites, opioid polymorphisms, that produce varied analgesic responses. These opioid polymorphisms may be responsible for some of the variations in pain relief and patient preferences for different opioid analgesics seen by clinicians.

Opioid Rotation

Patients with persistent pain may benefit from a technique called *opioid rotation* to provide adequate pain relief.[21] There are instances when upward titration of an opioid does not provide adequate pain relief or may produce untoward side effects. Using an opioid rotation technique can provide better pain relief for the patient. Simply put, this refers to switching to a different opioid analgesic which has the potential to decrease both pain intensity and unwanted side effects of the medication. The prescriber should use an equianalgesic chart such as the one provided below and should follow the formula provided.

To perform the opioid rotation, calculate the correct conversion of the medication using Table 2 and then decrease the new dose by 25% to 50% and offer adequate breakthrough medication.[33] The reduction in dose is needed because of the anticipated incomplete cross-tolerance (caused by the differences in mu receptor and binding) that may lead to greater effect and increased side effects if the dose were converted at full strength. Also consider the individual patient's comorbid health conditions and age.[33]

Table 2 Equianalgesic Table for Opioid Conversion

	Generic	Brand Name	Oral dose	Parenteral	
Immediate release	Morphine	Roxanol, MSIR	30 mg	10 mg	Relative potency 1:6 with acute dosing and 1:2 to 1:3 with chronic dosing
	Oxycodone	Roxicodone, Oxy IR	20 mg	NA	
	Hydromorphone	Dilaudid	7.5 mg	1.5 mg	
	Oxymorphone	Opana, Numorphan	10 mg	1 mg	Extended half-life with short-acting oral form
	Hydrocodone	Vicodin, Lortab	30 mg	NA	
	Fentanyl	Sublimaze	NA	100 μg	
	Methadone	Dolophine	5–10 mg	10 mg	Use with caution. Half-life of 12–150 hours accumulates with repeated dosing
	Meperidine	Demerol	NR	NR	Use with caution. Toxic metabolite normerperidine can cause seizures.

(continued)

Table 2 Continued

Controlled Release	Generic	Brand Name	Oral dose	Parenteral
Not recommended for opioid naïve patients	Morphine	MSContin, Avinza, Kadian	20–30 mg	
	Oxycodone	Oxycontin	20–30 mg	
	Fentanyl transdermal	Duragesic	NA	25 µg

Basic intravenous conversion: Morphine 1 mg = Dilaudid 0.2 mg; 0 mg = Dilaudid 0.2 mg = Fentanyl 10 µg

NR = not recommended

When switching from one opioid to another, reduce the dose by 25% to 50% with adequate breakthrough medication.

When switching to methadone, reduce the equianalgesic dose by 75% to 90%.

Breakthrough medication should be available when controlled release medications are being used.

All opioid medications should be carefully dosed and titrated with consideration for the individual patient and the medical condition of the patient.

Sources: Inturrisi C & Lipman A (2010) Bonica's management of Pain 1174–1175; Smith H & McCleane G (2009) Current Therapy in Pain Fine P & Portnoy R (2007) Opioid Analgesia; APS(2008) Principles of Analgesic Use in the Treatment of Acute Pain and Cancer Pain

Table 3 Medication Charts: Common Opioid Medications, Short Acting and Extended Release

Common Opioid Medications—Short Acting

Medication name	Generic name/combination name	Usual starting dose-Adults	Maximum dose
Codeine	Tylenol #3	30 to 60 mg by mouth every 4–6 hours	12 tablets in a 24-hour period Limited by acetaminophen dose; available as an elixir
Hydrocodone	Lortab	5 to 10 mg by mouth every 4–6 hours	Limited by acetaminophen dose
	Vicodin	5 to 10 mg by mouth every 6 hours	
Oxycodone	Percocet	5 mg every 6 hours	Limited by acetaminophen dose
Tramadol	Ultram	25 mg by mouth in AM	Maximum 400 mg per day
	Ultracet		Limited by acetaminophen dose
Tapentadol	Nucynta	50, 75, or 100 mg every 4–6 hours	No more than 700 mg on day 1 and thereafter 600 mg maximum
Oxymorphone	Opana	10–20 mg by mouth every 4 to 6 hours	

(continued)

Table 3 Continued

Common Opioid Medications—Short Acting

Medication name	Generic name/combination name	Usual starting dose-Adults	Maximum dose
Hydromorphone	Dilaudid	2 to 4 mg by mouth every 4 to 6 hours	Limited only by adverse side effects such as respiratory depression, sedation, nausea
Morphine	Morphine immediate release (MSIR)	5 to 15 mg by mouth every 4 hours	Limited by adverse side effects such as respiratory depression, sedation, nausea
	Roxanol	5 to 30 mg by mouth every 4 hours	
Methadone	Dolophine	2.5 to 10 mg by mouth every 3 to 4 hours	Use extreme care with dosing and medication initiation. Half-life ranges from 12 to 150 hours

* Acetaminophen dose should be limited to 4000 mg per day.
Medication information taken from Nursing 2010 Drug Handbook and Opioid Analgesics, Fine & Portnoy, 2007 and APS, 2008.

Common Opioid Medications – Extended Release

* Not intended to be crushed, chewed or used when alcohol is being ingested
** For use with opioid-tolerant patients on a scheduled basis, not prn

Medication	Generic name	Usual starting dose	Maximum dose
Morphine	Oramorph SR		
	Kadian	20 mg every 12 hours or 40 mg once daily	
	Avinza	20–30 mg by mouth daily	
	MS Contin	15 or 30 mg every 12 hours	
Oxycodone	Oxycontin	10 mg every 12 hours	
Oxymorphone	Opana ER	5 mg every 12 hours	
Tramadol	Ultram ER	100 mg once daily	300 mg per day
Dilaudid	Exalgo	8 mg to 64 mg daily converted from current opioid doses using Exalgo conversion equivalents: give 50% of converted daily dose give 50% of converted daily dose	

(continued)

Table 3 Continued

Common Opioid Medications—Extended Release

Medication	Generic name	Usual starting dose	Maximum dose
Morphine Sulfate with Naltrexone	Embeda	Convert the patient's total daily dose of current opioid and rescue dose by 50% when initiating therapy; dose every 12 hours	

Medication information taken from Nursing 2010 Drug Handbook and Opioid Analgesics; Fine & Portnoy, APS 2007; 2008; and PI for Exalgo, Embeda and Nucynta.

In order to be considered opioid-tolerant the patient should be taking at least 60 mg of oral morphine per day, 25 μg of fentanyl patch per hour, 30 mg of oxycodone per day, 8 mg of oral hydromorphone per day, or 25 mg of oral oxymorphone per day for a week or longer.

As an example of opioid rotation conversion: The patient is taking MS Contin 120 mg twice per day with MSIR 30 mg every 4 hours as needed for pain. The new medication is OxyContin. MS Contin 120 mg twice per day (240 mg/day) = OxyContin 80 mg twice per day (160 mg/day). MSIR 30 mg = oxycodone 20 mg every 4 hours. The new dose should be decreased by 25% to 50% to start and tritrated up if indicated.[21]

Adjusting Opioids for the Older Patient

In contrast to acetaminophen and NSAIDs, most opioids and tramadol are indicated for moderate to severe pain in older adults.[34] Specific recommendations for opioid use in older populations include lower doses (due to age-related decreases in creatinine clearance, liver size and function, glomerular filtration rate, muscle to fat ratio, and other metabolic changes with aging) and slower titration to reduce the onset of adverse events.[35] Special care must be taken to monitor for opioid-related adverse effects (e.g., sedation, confusion, and constipation), which may be more pronounced in older patients, particularly in those with cognitive impairment. A routine bowel monitoring and treatment regimen is recommended for older patients using long-term opioid therapy.[35]

Age-related changes relevant to opioid use include the following:

- Decreased renal clearance
- Decreased hepatic function
- Higher ratio of fat to lean muscle mass
- Decreased serum protein levels
- Reduced first-pass metabolism

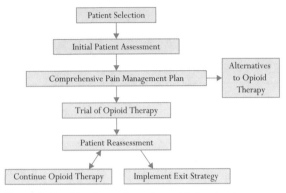

Figure 2 Algorithm for treating patients with chronic pain.
Source: Initiative on Pain Control. Opioid Analgesia Algorithm, 2004. www.painknowledge.org

Establishing baseline control with long-acting opioids as opposed to short-acting opioids in older persons may be more beneficial in the long run. However, aggressive titration or once-daily loading doses are not recommended because of the increased rate of adverse events. Around-the-clock medication administration can be helpful to both patient and caregiver when there are comorbid disabilities, particularly dementia or cognitive dysfunction, and dose administration is monitored. Lower doses of two synergistic agents may reduce dose-related adverse effects.

Because of the potential for drug–drug interactions, all patients on chronic pain medications should be asked about their use of over-the-counter products, vitamins, or herbal remedies. In addition, since older adults have a high prevalence of comorbid conditions requiring polypharmacy, a careful medication history should be taken to identify medications that alter CYP activity and may result in adverse drug reactions.

Using Opioids in Patients with a History of Substance Abuse

All patients have the right to have their pain assessed and treated. This includes some of the most difficult patients to treat: those with addictive disease or patients with a history of substance abuse. When opioids are provided to these patients, the prescriber should have careful documentation as to the pain complaint and the use of the medications solely for pain relief. A formal opioid agreement must be made and urine screens must be done on a random/intermittant basis. There should be only one prescriber, and the consequences of violating the agreement should be clearly stated and explained to the patient. These patients should also be in treatment with a substance abuse or mental health provider for additional support and coping skills training.

Patients with addiction disease or those with a history of substance abuse will need higher doses of medication to control pain, and using extended-release opioids can be helpful in maintaining a steady level of pain relief. Establishing a solid patient-provider relationship with mutual trust is critical to the success of any treatment plan.

Treating Opioid-Related Side Effects

V. DEVELOPING A COMPREHENSIVE TREATMENT AND MONITORING PLAN

A clinical guide for developing a comprehensive evaluation, treatment, and management plan for patients on chronic opioid therapy has several basic principles. The components are integrated below.

Table 4 Side Effects and Treatment

Side Effect	Treatment
Confusion	Lower dose; switch opioid
Constipation	Use traditional measures to treat constipation or switch opioids
Dizziness	Lower dose; add adjuvant medications
Edema and sweating	Switch opioids
Endocrine dysfunction, reduced libido, hypogonadism	Assess endocrine status at baseline and at least annually; consider opioid rotation, dose reduction, testosterone supplementation if hypogonadism is diagnosed; consider consultation with endocrinologist
Hives	Switch opioid; symptomatic treatment
Myoclonus	Switch opioids, or consider low-dose baclofen, clonazepam, or gabapentin
Nausea	Switch opioids; antiemetics
Pruritus	Switch opioids; antihistamines
Rash	Switch opioids; symptomatic treatment
Respiratory depression	"Start low, go slow"; close observation; supportive measures; naloxone for overdose with respiratory compromise
Sedation	Lower dose; adjuvant medications; add stimulants
Urinary retention	Switch opioids; lower dose
Vomiting	Switch opioids; co-prescribe antiemetics

Always check for other causes of these symptoms: they may not be due to opioid administration.

Table adapted from Pujol, LM, Katz, NP, and Zacharoff, KL (2007). The PainEDU.org Manual: A Clinical Companion, 3rd ed. Inflexxion, Inc. Newton, MA pages 123–127. Used with permission of Inflexxion, Inc.

Appropriate Diagnosis
- Obtain a complete history and physical focused on pain-related questions and assessment.
- Administer multidimensional pain assessment instruments.
- Review previous diagnostic studies and interventions.
- Review previous medication history and efficacy and side effects of medications.
- Identify coexisting medical conditions.
- Identify functional limitations.
- Order additional diagnostic studies if indicated.
- Conduct a psychological and opioid risk assessment (below).
- Consider appropriate differential diagnoses and assign pain diagnosis(es).

Psychological Assessment with Risk Assessment
- Assess personal history of psychiatric/mental health issues and treatments.
- Review personal history of illicit drug use/substance abuse.
- Review family history of illicit drug use/substance abuse and psychiatric history.
- Administer opioid risk screening instruments.
- Add psychiatric and/or opioid risk to diagnosis list if indicated.

Develop Treatment Plan
- Tailor the plan to the patient's pain condition and comorbidities (including mental health issues).
- Treatment may include pharmacological, behavioral, and rehabilitative domains.
- Include additional health practitioners in patient management as indicated.

- Based on your evaluation, determine if an opioid trial is indicated.
- Set mutual goals and expectations in all treatment domains.
- Discuss opioid exit strategy if goals are not met or the patient cannot adhere to safe opioid therapeutic management.
- Administer and discuss pre-opioid management tools, including opioid consent, opioid agreement, and baseline urine drug screen.

The patient's unique characteristics will help guide the treatment plan. For instance, if a patient has coexisting depression along with the pain syndrome, then a reasonable choice would be to include a tricyclic antidepressant or dual-uptake reuptake inhibitor antidepressants, which are also co-analgesic agents. Referral to a psychologist for treatment of depression or coping skills training would also be of benefit.

Once mutual treatment goals are set, it is important to discuss with the patient how the initial treatment plan will be altered. This may include discontinuing opioid therapy and using a non-opioid analgesic if treatment goals are not met after a reasonable trial of medication or if the patient has difficulty adhering to safe practices associated with opioid use.

Informed Consent

Obtaining an informed consent in the setting of opioid analgesic management for persistent pain involves the same principles as in other medical settings. It is a process of communication between patient and clinician that results in the patient's agreement to undergo a specific medical intervention. This discussion should be conducted by the treating clinician and should include:

- Diagnosis
- Purpose of proposed treatment
- Risks
- Benefits
- Alternatives
- Expectations

Opioid Treatment Agreement

For patients on long-term opioid therapy, a treatment agreement is a useful tool to make clear the expected patient responsibilities that accompany opioid management. The agreement serves as an educational tool for the patient and can be revisited intermittently throughout the course of opioid therapy to reinforce the importance of its terms. The agreement should be signed by the patient and a copy given to the patient. If the patient is being treated by a pain specialist, a copy should also be sent to the patient's primary provider. Key elements of an opioid treatment agreement may include:

- Only one clinician to prescribe pain medicines
- Use of a single pharmacy
- Patient should take the medication as prescribed (no dose escalations, sharing, or altering medication).
- Refills should be obtained at prearranged intervals (no early, weekend, or night refills).
- Intermittent urine screens and/or pill counts.
- Patient should not use illicit substances.
- Patient should safeguard opioids from loss or theft.

OAPN

CONSENT FOR CHRONIC OPIOID THERAPY

A consent form from the **American Academy of Pain Medicine**

Dr. _____ is prescribing opioid medicine, sometimes called narcotic analgesics, to me for a diagnosis of_____.

This decision was made because my condition is serious or other treatments have not helped my pain.

I am aware that the use of such medicine has certain risks associated with it, including, but not limited to: sleepiness or drowsiness, constipation, nausea, itching, vomiting, dizziness, allergic reaction, slowing of breathing rate, slowing of reflexes or reaction time, physical dependence, tolerance to analgesia, addiction, and the possibility that the medicine will not provide complete pain relief.

I am aware of the possible risks and benefits of other types of treatments that do not involve the use of opioids. The other treatments discussed included:

_____

_____

_____

I will tell my doctor about all other medicines and treatments that I am receiving.

I will not be involved in any activity that may be dangerous to me or someone else if I feel drowsy or am not thinking clearly. I am aware that even if I do not notice it, my reflexes and reaction time might still be slowed.

Such activities include, but are not limited to: using heavy equipment or a motor vehicle, working in unprotected heights, or being responsible for another individual who is unable to care for himself or herself.

I am aware that certain other medicines such as nalbuphine (Nubain™), pentazocine (Talwin™), buprenorphine (Buprenex™), and butorphanol (Stadol™), may reverse the action of the medicine I am using for pain control. Taking any of these other medicines while I am taking my pain medicines can cause symptoms like a bad flu, called a withdrawal syndrome. I agree not to take any of these medicines and to tell any other doctors that I am taking an opioid as my pain medicine and cannot take any of the medicines listed above.

I am aware that addiction is defined as the use of a medicine even if it causes harm, having cravings for a drug, feeling the need to use a drug and a decreased quality of life. I am aware that the chance of becoming addicted to my pain medicine is very low. I am aware that the development of addiction has been reported rarely in medical journals and is much more common in a person who has a family or personal history of addiction. I agree to tell my doctor my complete and honest personal drug history and that of my family to the best of my knowledge.

I understand that physical dependence is a normal, expected result of using these medicines for a long time. I understand that physical dependence is not the same as addiction. I am aware physical dependence means that if my pain medicine use is markedly decreased, stopped, or reversed by some of the agents mentioned above, I will

(continued)

experience a withdrawal syndrome. This means I may have any or all of the following: runny nose, yawning, large pupils, goose bumps, abdominal pain and cramping, diarrhea, irritability, aches throughout my body, and a flu-like feeling. I am aware that opioid withdrawal is uncomfortable but not life threatening.

I am aware that tolerance to analgesia means that I may require more medicine to get the same amount of pain relief. I am aware that tolerance to analgesia does not seem to be a big problem for most patients with chronic pain, however, it has been seen and may occur in me. If it occurs, increasing doses may not always help and may cause unacceptable side effects. Tolerance or failure to respond well to opioids may cause my doctor to choose another form of treatment.

(**Males only**) I am aware that chronic opioid use has been associated with low testosterone levels in males. This may affect my mood, stamina, sexual desire, and physical and sexual performance. I understand that my doctor may check my blood to see if my testosterone level is normal.

(**Females Only**) If I plan to become pregnant or believe that I have become pregnant while taking this pain medicine, I will immediately call my obstetric doctor and this office to inform them. I am aware that, should I carry a baby to delivery while taking these medicines, the baby will be physically dependent upon opioids. I am aware that the use of opioids is not generally associated with a risk of birth defects. However, birth defects can occur whether or not the mother is on medicines and there is always the possibility that my child will have a birth defect while I am taking an opioid.

> I had read this form or had it read to me. I understand all of it. I have had a chance to have all of my questions regarding this treatment answered to my satisfaction. By signing this form voluntarily, I give my consent for the treatment of my pain with opioid pain medicines.
>
> Patient signature _____ Date _____
>
> Witness to above _____
>
> *Approved by the AAPM Executive Committee on January 14, 1999.*
>
> "Consent for Chronic Opioid Therapy" is a copyrighted work of the American Academy of Pain Medicine. © 1999 American Academy of Pain Medicine. Reprinted with permission.

Urine Drug Testing

Urine drug testing (UDT) should be used in conjunction with opioid agreements and the patient assessment and documentation principles. UDT can detect the presence of a prescribed drug and/or its metabolites and the presence of illicit substances. In the clinic, UDT is used to support treatment decisions and to assist in monitoring and diagnosis of drug misuse or addiction. Generally this type of testing is considered to be the most effective biologically based method for determining the presence or absence of most drugs. It has 1- to 3-day window of detection for most drugs and can detect parent drug and/or its metabolite(s) and thus can demonstrate recent use of prescription medications (e.g., opioids, benzodiazepines, amphetamines, barbiturates) and illegal substances (e.g., heroin, cocaine, marijuana, phencyclidine). However, some caution must be used in interpreting results. For example, not all substances can be detected, and false-positive and false-negative results and misinterpretations are common. Potential confounding metabolic and technical factors exist as well.

General guidelines in UDT include:

- Ensure proper collection, handling, and documentation of the specimen.
- Know the appropriate tests to order and how to interpret the results.
- Be prepared to address unanticipated results.
- Document discussion of UDT results with the patient (both anticipated and unanticipated).

A common practice is to initially test all patients who are starting opioid therapy and then test intermittently throughout the course of treatment. The frequency of retesting can be determined by office policy or risk stratification. In some practices, it may be easier to set a policy that patients are tested every 3 months. Nurse practitioners may identify a patient at greater risk for misuse as determined by PADT, COMM, or aberrant behaviors; under these circumstances more frequent vigilance is warranted.

Several methods are available for urine drug testing. **Qualitative** tests indicate the presence or absence of drug and include point-of-care testing (POCT) and enzyme immunoassay (EIA, ELISA). **Quantitative** results, expressed in ng/mL, include fluorescence polarization immunoassay (FPIA), gas chromatography/mass spectrometry (GC/MS), and high-performance liquid chromatography/mass spectrometry (HPLC/MS).

Testing procedures vary from laboratory to laboratory but should include a two-step process. The first step is immunoassay testing, which is designed to classify substances as either present or absent. Immunoassays are rapid tests and may detect either specific drugs or classes of drugs. The ability to detect a drug by this method is determined by the drug concentration in the urine and the assay's cutoff level.

Immunoassays are also subject to reactivity, so it is possible for a drug with a similar chemical compound to appear positive for the drug being tested for. For example, standard test for opioids are highly effective for picking up morphine and codeine, but may not distinguish which one is present. Similarly, semisynthetic or synthetic opioids such as oxycodone or fentanyl might not be detected, even though they are present.[37]

The second, or confirmatory, step in UDT is GC/MS or HPLC. This method confirms the presence of specific drugs as well as their metabolites. The results must be interpreted carefully. The presence of specific opioid metabolites may be reported as a drug not prescribed, and this requires careful interpretation. For example, codeine metabolizes to morphine, so both substances may be identified in urine following codeine use. Hydrocodone can be metabolized to hydromorphone. It is important not to jump to conclusions if you are not familiar with drug metabolic pathways or the potential for cross-reactivity. Most reputable UDT companies have pharmacologists available to assist in interpreting results.

Retention of drug in the urine is based on time of last drug use, variability of urine specimens, the drug's metabolism and half-life, the patient's physical condition and fluid intake, and the method and frequency of ingestion. The following general guidelines may be helpful in UDT interpretation when taken together with the factors previously mentioned.

A positive UDT result is defined as the prescribed drug not present, presence of an unprescribed opioid, or the presence

Table 5 Drug Test Quick-Reference Guide

DRUG	DETECTION TIME IN URINE	DETECTION & POSITIVE TEST RESULT COMMENTS
AMPHETAMINE CLASS		
Amphetamine	3–5 days	**Positive Test:** Tests negative for methamphetamine. Prescribed as Adderall®, Dexedrine®.
Amphetamine Methamphetamine	3–5 days	**Positive Test:** Evidence of having taken some form of methamphetamine, not necessarily illicit. Prescription methamphetamine includes Desoxyn®, or metabolites of Didrex® and Selegiline®. If IA is positive and MS is negative, this could indicate use of amphetamine class drug which is not amphetamine or methamphetamine. Examples are phentermine or MDMA (ecstasy), or a high amount of ephedrine/pseudoephedrine/ephedra, or something unidentifiable triggering a positive.
BARBITURATES		**Detection:** Detection time depends on the dose, frequency, and specific barbiturate.
Butalbital	4–6 days	Commonly prescribed as Fiorinal® or Fioricet®.
Pentobarbital	4–6 days	Prescribed as Nembutal®.
Phenobarbital	Up to 16 days	Prescribed as Luminal®. Phenobarbital is also a metabolite of primidone (Mysoline®).
Secobarbital	4–6 days	Prescribed as Seconal®.

BENZODIAZEPINES		
Alprazolam	2–4 days	**Positive Test:** If IA is positive and MS is negative, this could indicate use of a benzodiazepine not covered by the MS confirmation (e.g., Clonazepam), an additive response from parent and/or metabolites that individually are below the MS cutoff, or an undetermined urine component triggering an IA response but not affecting MS results.
Clonazepam	See Comments	**Positive Test:** Presence of Alprazolam and/or its metabolite, Alphahydroxyalprazolam indicates use of alprazolam (Xanax®). **Detection:** Heat and light sensitive; not currently included in the MS confirmation panel.
Diazepam	See Nordiazepam and Oxazepam	**Detection:** Ameritox tests for 2 metabolites of diazepam, nordiazepam, and oxazepam.
Lorazepam	5–7 days	**Detection:** Cross-reactivity of IA reagents with lorazepam is limited. MS testing is available with a higher sensitivity to lorazepam.
Nordiazepam	2–4 days	**Positive Test:** Indicates use of a benzodiazepine class drug, which could include, but is not limited to, Valium®, Librium®, or Tranxene®.
Oxazepam	2–7 days	**Detection:** Presence of only oxazepam could indicate it has been several days since the last dose of a benzodiazepine class drug including, but not limited to, Valium®, Librium®, Tranxene®, or use of the drugs Restoril® or Serax®.

(continued)

Table 5 Continued

DRUG	DETECTION TIME IN URINE	DETECTION & POSITIVE TEST RESULT COMMENTS
BENZOYLECGONINE	2–3 days	Benzoylecgonine is a metabolite specific to cocaine. Similar sounding drugs such as Novocaine® or lidocaine will not produce this result.
BUPRENORPHINE	2–4 days	**Detection:** May be detectable longer, depending on dose. Prescribed as Suboxone®.
CARISOPRODOL Meprobamate	24–48 hours 24–48 hours	**Detection:** Very low levels excreted in urine, Rx Guardian monitoring measures the major metabolite, Meprobamate. Prescribed as Soma®. Metabolite of carisoprodol, or can be prescribed as Equanil® or Miltown®.
COTININE	7–10 days	**Detection:** Dependent on the initial level of cotinine and time since cessation of smoking.
ETHANOL Ethyl Glucuronide Ethyl Sulfate	Up to 24 hours 3–5 days	**Positive Test:** Result of glucose/yeast analysis must be noted as ethanol and can be produced post-collection in their presence. **Positive Test:** Biomarkers have good specificity for alcohol ingestion.

FENTANYL AND NORFENTANYL	1–3 days	**Positive Test:** Presence of Fentanyl or its metabolite Norfentanyl indicates use of a fentanyl product. Prescribed as Actiq®, Duragesic®, or Fentora®.
GABAPENTIN	2–4 days	**Detection:** Dependent on dose. Prescribed as Neurontin®.
HEROIN METABOLITE (6-MAM)	Up to 24 hours	**Positive Test:** The presence of 6-MAM indicates recent use of heroin.
MEPERIDINE	24–48 hours	**Positive Test:** Presence of meperidine and its metabolite. Normeperidine indicates use of meperidine product. Prescribed as Demerol®.
MARIJUANA Infrequent User	3–5 days	**Detection:** Neither the medication Protonix® nor second-hand smoke will likely produce a positive result.
Frequent User	Up to 14 days	**Detection:** Neither the medication Protonix® nor second-hand smoke will likely produce a positive result.
Chronic User	Up to 30–45 days	**Detection:** Neither the medication Protonix® nor second-hand smoke will likely produce a positive result.

(continued)

Table 5 Continued

DRUG	DETECTION TIME IN URINE	DETECTION & POSITIVE TEST RESULT COMMENTS
METHADONE	Up to 14 days	**Positive Test:** Presence of methadone or its metabolite EDDPI indicates use of methadone product. Prescribed as Methadone, Methadose, or Dolophine.
METHYLPHENIDATE	24–48 hours	**Positive Test:** Presence of Ritalinic Acid (metabolite) indicates use of methylphenidate. Prescribed as Ritalin® and Concerta®.
OPIATES	2–3 days	**Positive Test:** If IA is positive and MS is negative, this could indicate use of an opiate not covered by the MS confirmation panel (e.g., dihydrocodeine); an additive response from parent and metabolites that individually are below the MS cutoff; or an undetermined urine component triggering an IA response but not affecting MS results. **Positive Test:** Indicates ingestion of codeine and/or morphine.
Codeine and Morphine	2–3 days	A small percentage of the population exhibits poor metabolism of codeine to morphine.
Morphine Only	2–3 days	**Positive Test:** Can result from the following: codeine, heroin, morphine, or poppy seeds (when morphine concentrations are relatively low). A small percentage of morphine can metabolize to hydromorphone. Please contact an Ameritox Toxicology Specialist℠ to discuss.

Hydrocodone and Hydromorphone	2–3 days	**Positive Test:** Evidence of hydrocodone use within 2–3 days. Note: A small percentage of the population exhibits poor metabolism of hydrocodone into hydromorphone. A positive hydrocodone value and negative hydromorphone could be due to individual metabolism, evidence that the patient took hydrocodone immediately prior to collection, or hydromorphone level is too low to detect.
Hydromorphone Only	2–3 days	**Positive Test:** May result from Dilaudid®; or low levels may be due to hydrocodone metabolism. High levels of morphine can cause low levels of hydromorphone.
Oxycodone and/or Oxymorphone and/or Noroxycodone Oxymorphone Only	2–3 days	**Positive Test:** Evidence of oxycodone use within 2–3 days. Positive Test: Low levels could be due to oxycodone metabolism or can come from Opana®.
PCP	Up to 10 days	PCP = Phencyclidine. This is an illicit drug.
PREGABALIN	24–48 hours	**Positive Test:** Presence of Pregabalin indicates use of pregabalin product. Prescribed as Lyrica®.
PROPOXYPHENE	Up to 7 days	**Positive Test:** Presence of Propoxyphene or its metabolite.
Propoxyphene or Norpoxyphene	Up to 7 days	Norpoxyphene indicates use of propoxyphene product. Positive for norpoxyphene but negative for propoxyphene is evidence of use within 7 days. Prescribed as Darvon® or Darvocet®.

(continued)

Table 5 Continued

DRUG	DETECTION TIME IN URINE	DETECTION & POSITIVE TEST RESULT COMMENTS
TAPENTADOL	1–2 days	**Positive Test:** Presence of Tapentadol or its metabolite N-desmethyltapentadol indicates use of Tapentadol product. Prescribed as Nucynta®.
TRAMADOL	2–4 days	**Positive Test:** Presence of Tramadol or its metabolite O-desmethyltramadol indicates use of Tramadol product. Prescribed as Ultram®, Ultracet or Ryzolt™.

Key: IA = Immunoassay; MS = Mass Spectrometry

Reprinted with permission. © 2010, Ameritox, Ltd. All rights reserved. AMERITOX, the AMERITOX logos, PAIN MEDICATION MONITORING SOLUTIONS, AMERITOX MEDICATION MONITORING SOLUTIONS, Rx Guardian Autoreminder, Rx Guardian and PROTECT YOUR PATIENTS, PROTECT YOUR PRACTICE, are trademarks of Ameritox. All other trademarks are the claimed trademarks of others. ATX 1008-1002 February 2010.

of an illicit substance. At the onset, none of these should mandate immediate dismissal from the clinic. The most concerning of these is the absence of the prescribed opioid, which may represent diversion of the drug. Consider the possibilities that the patient may not have recently used the medication, the patient is a rapid metabolizer, the test was not sensitive enough to detect concentrations, or there were lab/clerical errors. In these instances, a second UDT may be needed for clarification. If these explanations do not seem reasonable, discharge from the clinic may be warranted to reduce the risk of drug diversion.

Reassessment

Reassessment on a regular basis should include evaluation of pain, function, the effect of pain on well-being and quality of life, and achievement of treatment goals. Pharmacological regimens should be individualized, and frequent comprehensive assessment should provide the rationale for continued therapy, a modification in therapy, and assessment of aberrant behaviors. For example, some patients may report that their pain intensity has decreased to an acceptable level, yet the medication regimen induces excessive sedation that decreases the patient's ability to function. In this case, adjustments to the pharmacological regimen are necessary, and a less sedating medication or nonpharmacologic treatment should be added. On the other hand, if the treatment goals are being met, and no adverse medication effects or aberrant behaviors are noted, then the treatment plan should be continued.

During the initial titration phase, assessment is scheduled on a more frequent basis (weekly or every other week) to review for efficacy and potential side effects and to provide continued education. Once an effective dose is stabilized, monthly visits may be scheduled.

A useful mnemonic device to assess pain-related outcome in all domains of pain management is "the four A's for pain management":[38]

- **Analgesia:** may use a visual analog scale or other instrument to assess pain intensity. This outcome may not be the most important or the one with the most dramatic change for patients with persistent pain.
- **Activities of Daily Living:** assess quality-of-life issues and functionality
- **Adverse Events:** assess for adverse side effects associated with the use of opioid analgesics and other medications. Routine assessment for constipation in essential.
- **Aberrant Drug-Taking Behavior:** assess for signs outside the acceptable parameters for opioid therapy, such as multiple episodes of prescription "loss," concurrent abuse of related illicit drugs, multiple dose escalations despite warnings, and repeated episodes of gross impairment or dishevelment.

When managing patients on opioid therapy, additional tools for assessment and documentation may be helpful. The PADT is a specialized chart note designed to aid healthcare providers in monitoring outcomes during long-term therapy for non-cancer patients on opioid therapy. It takes only minutes to complete and should supplement existing documentation. The elements of the 4A's are the foundation of the tool, and a final section requires the interpretation of the data to formulate an assessment of the risks (e.g., side effects) and benefits (pain relief, improved functioning) of continued therapy and designation of the analgesic plan (continued therapy, dose adjustment, discontinuation).[34]

SAFE OPIOID PRESCRIBING FOR NURSE PRACTITIONERS

PROGRESS NOTE
Pain Assessment and Documentation Tool (PADT™)

Patient Name: _____

Record #: _____

Assessment Date: _____

Patient Stamp Here

Current Analgesic Regimen			
Drug name	Strength (e.g., mg)	Frequency	Maximum Total Daily Dose

The PADT is a clinician-directed interview; that is, the clinician asks the questions, and the clinician records the responses. The Analgesia, Activities of Daily Living, and Adverse Events sections may be completed by the physician, nurse practitioner, physician assistant, or nurse. The Potential Aberrant Drug-Related Behavior and Assessment sections must be completed by the physician. Ask the patient the questions below, except as noted.

Analgesia

If zero indicates "no pain" and ten indicates "pain as bad as it can be," on a scale of 0 to 10, what is your level of pain for the following questions?

1. What was your pain level on average during the past week? (Please circle the appropriate number.)
   No Pain 0 1 2 3 4 5 6 7 8 9 10 **Pain as bad as it can be**

2. What was your pain level at its worst during the past week?
   No Pain 0 1 2 3 4 5 6 7 8 9 10 **Pain as bad as it can be**

3. What percentage of your pain has been relieved during the past week? (Write in a percentage between 0% and 100%.) _____

4. Is the amount of pain relief you are now obtaining from your current pain reliever(s) enough to make a real difference in your life?
   ☐ Yes   ☐ No

5. **Query to clinician**: Is the patient's pain relief clinically significant?
   ☐ Yes   ☐ No   ☐ Unsure

(continued)

Activities of Daily Living

Please indicate whether the patient's functioning with the current pain reliever(s) is Better, the Same, or Worse since the patient's last assessment with the PADT.* (Please check the box for Better, Same, or Worse for each item below.)

	Better	Same	Worse
1. Physical functioning	☐	☐	☐
2. Family relationships	☐	☐	☐
3. Social relationships	☐	☐	☐
4. Mood	☐	☐	☐
5. Sleep patterns	☐	☐	☐
6. Overall functioning	☐	☐	☐

* If the patient is receiving his or her first PADT assessment, the clinician should compare the patient's functional status with other reports from the last office visit.

Adverse Events

1. Is patient experiencing any side effects from current pain reliever(s)?
   ☐ Yes ☐ No

Ask patient about potential side effects:

	None	Mild	Moderate	Severe
a. Nausea	☐	☐	☐	☐
b. Vomiting	☐	☐	☐	☐
c. Constipation	☐	☐	☐	☐
d. Itching	☐	☐	☐	☐
f. Sweating	☐	☐	☐	☐
g. Fatigue	☐	☐	☐	☐
h. Drowsiness	☐	☐	☐	☐
i. Other _____		☐	☐	☐
j. Other _____		☐	☐	☐

2. Patient's overall severity of side effects?

   ☐ None   ☐ Mild   ☐ Moderate   ☐ Severe

SAFE OPIOID PRESCRIBING
FOR NURSE PRACTITIONERS

Potential Aberrant Drug-Related Behavior
This section must be completed by the <u>physician</u>.

*Please **check** any of the following items that you discovered during your interactions with the patient. Please note that some of these are directly observable (e.g., appears intoxicated), while others may require more active listening and/or probing. Use the "Assessment" section below to note additional details.*

- ☐ Purposeful over-sedation
- ☐ Negative mood change
- ☐ Appears intoxicated
- ☐ Increasingly unkempt or impaired
- ☐ Involvement in car or other accident
- ☐ Requests frequent early renewals
- ☐ Increased dose without authorization
- ☐ Reports lost or stolen prescriptions
- ☐ Attempts to obtain prescriptions from other doctors
- ☐ Changes route of administration
- ☐ Uses pain medication in response to situational stressor
- ☐ Insists on certain medications by name
- ☐ Contact with street drug culture
- ☐ Abusing alcohol or illicit drugs
- ☐ Hoarding (i.e., stockpiling) of medication
- ☐ Arrested by police
- ☐ Victim of abuse

Other: _____
_____
_____

(continued)

OAPN

Assessment: (This section must be completed by the <u>physician</u>.)
Is your overall impression that this patient is benefiting (i.e., benefits, such as pain relief, outweigh side effects) from opioid therapy? ☐ Yes ☐ No ☐ Unsure
Comments: _____
Specific Analgesic Plan:
☐ Continue present regimen　　　　Comments: _____
☐ Adjust dose of present analgesic
☐ Switch analgesics
☐ Add/Adjust concomitant therapy
☐ Discontinue/taper off opioid therapy
Date: _____　　Physician's signature: _____
Provided as a service to the medical community by Janssen Pharmaceutica Products, L.P. Reprinted with permission.

Unmet Treatment Goals and Exit Strategy

Evaluation of initial and ongoing treatment goals is part of the comprehensive management plan. This is especially challenging when patients are managed on opioid therapy as part of the plan. Patients who are compliant, with satisfactory pain and function goals, may be managed on opioid therapy indefinitely as long as there are no adverse side effects. If this is not the case, an exit strategy for discontinuation of opioids must be employed. After thorough evaluation, consider the following strategies:

- Continue nonopioid pharmacological treatment after supported titration off opioid analgesia.
- Refer the patient to an addiction specialist.
- Restructure the treatment plan for closer monitoring of aberrant behavior.

- Continue treatment contingent upon patient participation in physical rehabilitation, cognitive-behavioral strategies, and/or mental health counseling.
- Discharge the patient from the practice with referral sources for appropriate treatment.

Documentation

The importance of documentation cannot be stressed enough. It must be thorough and continuous. Pain management decision points must be supported by patient assessment features. The various instruments provided in this book may assist in this process.

VI. INTEGRATING COMPLEMENTARY METHODS INTO THE TREATMENT PLAN

Nonpharmacological modalities can be useful in the treatment of pain syndromes, either on their own or as adjuncts to pharmacotherapy. For example, physical therapy, transcutaneous electrical nerve stimulation, hypnosis, meditation, relaxation, guided imagery, biofeedback, prayer, and music therapy have all demonstrated some efficacy in relieving subjective pain complaints. Therefore, integrating complementary medicine into the care of patients with pain syndromes has the potential to yield promising results.

The National Center for Complementary and Alternative Medicine (NCCAM) defines complementary and alternative medicine as

> "a group of diverse medical and health care systems, practices, and products that are not presently considered to be part of conventional medicine. Complementary medicine is used *together with* conventional medicine; alternative medicine is used *in place of* conventional medicine."[c]

Four distinct types of complementary and alternative medicine domains have been defined by NCCAM: (1) biologically based therapies, which use substances found in nature, such as herbs, special diets, or vitamins; (2) mind-body medicine, which uses a variety of techniques designed to enhance the mind's ability to affect bodily function and symptoms, such as cognitive-behavioral therapies, meditation, guided imagery, and prayer; (3) manipulative and body-based practices that are based on manipulation or movement of one or more body parts, including massage, chiropractic manipulation, and reflexology; and (4) energy medicine, which involves the use of energy fields, such as magnetic fields or biofields.

Questions to Consider for Complementary and Alternative Medicine Use

- Has the conventional medical evaluation been completed?
- What is the diagnosis?
- What are the conventional treatment options?
- Have the conventional treatment options been tried? Refused? Exhausted?
- What is the chief symptom intended for treatment by complementary and alternative medicine?
- What are the complementary and alternative medicine preferences of the patient?
- Are there safety and efficacy data supporting the use of the complementary and alternative medicine being considered?
- Are there identified patient barriers for the use of the specific complementary and alternative medicine?

(Adapted from Bruckenthal P. Integrating nonpharmacologic and alternative strategies into a comprehensive management approach for older adults with pain. *Pain Manag Nurs* 2010;11:523–531.)

NOTES

A. Krantz, M., et al. (2009) QTc Interval Screening in Methadone Treatment. Annals of Internal Medicine. 150: 387–395.
B. Janssen prescribing information, available at www.Janssen.com
C. NCCAM. What is CAM? http://nccam.nih.gov/health/whatiscam/overview.htm

REFERENCES

1. *VA/DoD clinical practice guidelines for the management of opioid therapy for chronic pain.* (2003) Available at www.guideline.gov
2. Wilson P, Caplan R, Connis R, et al. Practice guidelines for chronic pain management: A report by the American Society of Anesthesiologists task force on pain management, chronic pain section. *Anesthesiology* 1997;86(4):995–1004.
3. Chou R, Fanciullo G, Fine P, et al. Clinical guidelines for the use of opioids therapy in chronic noncancer pain. *J Pain* 2009;10(2):113–130.
4. Trescot A, Helm S, Hansen H, et al. Opioids in the management of chronic non-cancer pain: An update from the American Society of Interventional Pain Physicians' (ASIPP) Guidelines. *Pain Physician* 2008;11:S5–S62.
5. American Academy of Pain Medicine and American Pain Society. *The use of opioids for the treatment of chronic pain.* Glenview, IL: APS, 1997.
6. American Academy of Pain Medicine, American Pain Society, American Society of Addiction Medicine (2004). *Public policy statement on the rights and responsibilities of healthcare professionals in the use of opioids for the treatment of pain.*
7. American Geriatrics Society Panel on the Pharmacological Management of Persistent Pain in Older Persons. Pharmacological management of persistent pain in older persons. *J Am Geriatrics Soc* 2009;57(8):1331–1346.

8. Stanos S, Fishbain D, Fishman S. Pain management with opioid analgesics: Balancing risk and benefit. *Phys Med Rehab* 2009; 88(3):S69–S99.

9. Flemming MF, Balousek SL, Klessig CL, Mundt MP, Brown DD. Substance abuse disorders in a primary care sample receiving daily opioid therapy. *J Pain* 2007;8(7):573–582.

10. Fishbain DA, Cole B, Lewis J, Rosamoff H, Rosamoff R. What percentage of chronic nonmalignant pain patients exposed chronic opioid analgesic therapy develop abuse/addiction and or aberrant drug-related behaviors? A structured evidence-based review. *Pain Med* 2008;79(4):444–459.

11. LaGangna ML, Monmanney T. Doctor found liable in suit over pain. *Los Angeles Times*, June 15, 2001:A1, A34.

12. Yi M. Doctor found reckless for not relieving pain. *San Francisco Chronicle* June 15, 2001: A1, A18.

13. D'Arcy Y. Be in the know about pain management. *Nurse Practitioner* 2009;34(4):43–47.

14. Ciphers DJ, Hooker RS, Guerra P. Prescribing trends by nurse practitioners and physician assistants in the United States. *J Am Acad Nurse Practitioners* 2006;18:291–296.

15. Olsen Y, Admit G, Ford D. Opioid prescribing by US primary care physicians from 1992 to 2001. *J Pain* 2006;7(4):225–235.

16. McCarberg B, Stanos S, D'Arcy Y. *Low back and neck pain.* Oxford University Press, 2009.

17. Weiner DK, Herr K. Comprehensive assessment & interdisciplinary treatment planning: an integrative overview. In: Weiner DK, Herr K, Rudy TE, eds. *Persistent pain in older adults: an interdisciplinary guide for treatment*. Springer Publishing Company, 2002.

18. D'Arcy Y. Chapter 13: Pain assessment. In: *American Society of Pain Management Nurses core curriculum*. Kendall Hunt Professional, 2009.

19. Butler S, Busman S, Fernandex K, Jamison R. Validation of a screener and opioids assessment measure for patients with chronic pain. *Pain* 2004;112:65–75.

20. Passik S, et al. Addiction-related assessment tools and pain management instruments for a screening, treatment planning, and monitoring compliance. *Pain Medicine* 2008;9(S2):S145–S166.

21. D'Arcy Y. *Compact clinical guide to chronic pain: An evidence based approach*. New York: Springer, 2010.

22. American Pain Society, American Academy of Pain Medicine, American Society of Addiction Medicine. *Definitions related to the use of opioids for the treatment of pain*. 2001.

23. Fine P, Portnoy R. *A clinical guide to opioid analgesia*. Vendome Group, Healthcare Division, 2007.

24. Buppert C. The legal pitfalls in prescribing opioids. *Topics in Advanced Practice Nursing e-Journal*. Listed Nov. 18, 2009. Available at www.medscape.com, Article 712414.

25. McCarberg B, Stanos S, D'Arcy Y. *Low back and neck pain*. New York: Oxford University Press, 2010.

26. American Pain Society. *Principles of analgesic use in the treatment of acute pain and cancer pain*. Glenview, IL: APS, 2008.

27. D'Arcy Y. *Pain management: evidence-based tools and techniques for nursing pofessionals*. Marblehead, MA: HcPro, 2007.

28. *Nursing 2010 drug handbook*. Philadelphia: Lippincott Williams & Wilkins, 2009.

29. Adams M, Pieniaszek H, Gammaitoni A, Ahdieh H. Oxymorphone extended release does not affect CYP2C9 or CYP34A metabolic pathways. *J Clin Pharmacol* 2005;45:337–345.

30. Adams M, Ahdieh H. Pharmacokinetics and dose proportionality of oxymorphone extended release and its metabolites: Results of a randomized crossover study. *Pharmacotherapy* 2004;24(4):468–476.

31. Katz N, McCarber B, Eisner L. *Managing chronic pain with opioids in primary care.* Newton, MA: Inflexxion, 2007.
32. D'Arcy Y. Avoid the dangers of opioid therapy. *American Nurse Today* 2009;4(5):16–22.
33. Indelicato RA, Portnoy R. Opioid rotation in the management of refractory cancer pain. *J Clin Oncol* 2002;20(1):348–352.
34. Pharmacological management of persistent pain in older persons. *J Am Geriatr Soc* 2009;57(8):1331–1346.
35. Pergolizzi J, Boger RH, Budd K, Dahan A, Erdine S, Hans G, et al. Opioids and the management of chronic severe pain in the elderly: consensus statement of an International Expert Panel with focus on the six clinically most often used World Health Organization Step III opioids (buprenorphine, fentanyl, hydromorphone, methadone, morphine, oxycodone). *Pain Pract* 2008;8(4):287–313.
36. Gourlay DL, Heit HA, Almahrezi A. Universal precautions in pain medicine: a rational approach to the treatment of chronic pain. *Pain Med* 2005;6(2):100–112.
37. Gourlay D, Heit H, Caplan Y. *Urine drug testing in clinical practice: Dispelling the myths and designing strategies.* Stamford, CT: PharmaCom Group, Inc., 2004.
38. Passik SD, Kirsh KL, Whitcomb L, Portenoy RK, Katz NP, Kleinman L, et al. A new tool to assess and document pain outcomes in chronic pain patients receiving opioid therapy. *Clin Ther* 2004;26(4):552–561.